Tiny Bites

Tiny Bites

A Guide to Gastric Surgery for the Morbidly Obese

Saundra Beauchamp-Parke

Jessica Kingsley Publishers
London and New York

First published in the United Kingdom in 2002 by
Jessica Kingsley Publishers Ltd,
116 Pentonville Road,
London N1 9JB, England
and
29 West 35th Street, 10th fl.
New York, NY 10001–2299, USA.

www.jkp.com

Copyright © 2002 Saundra Beauchamp-Parke

Printed digitally since 2004

Library of Congress Cataloging in Publication Data
A CIP catalog record for this book is available from the Library of Congress

British Library Cataloguing in Publication Data
A CIP catalogue record for this book is available from the British Library

ISBN 1 84310 704 X

Contents

Foreword

There is an epidemic of obesity afflicting industrialized societies throughout the globe, nowhere better exemplified than in the USA where obesity has increased by more than twenty-five per cent in the last three decades. In the USA 300,000 people die annually of obesity related disease, with direct and indirect costs to society amounting to $99.2 billion in 1995, approximating ten per cent of the national healthcare budget. This is in spite of a diet industry which encouraged the populace to expend $33 billion annually in weight loss endeavors in the early 1990s and the *Healthy People 2000* government-sponsored campaign in 1990, one of the goals of which was to reduce the prevalence of overweight people. Obesity in the United States has increased progressively and is now at an all time high. This trend, alarmingly, even affects children, a fact which bodes ill for future generations.

The population most severely afflicted by this disease are termed 'morbidly obese' and they not only suffer the miseries of extreme obesity, in terms of physical discomfort, social discrimination and emotional distress, but are also subject to life threatening disease processes such as adult onset diabetes, high blood pressure, coronary heart disease, stroke, several forms of cancer, sleep apnea[1] and sudden death.

Attempts to stay the rising tide of obesity in the population seem to have been unsuccessful, with a single exception, namely, the use of surgery. Over the past forty years the concept of influence over nutrition by surgical means has evolved from that of an empirical and inexact experiment to its current status as a widely accepted, practical method of control of overweight's most life-threatening manifestation, morbid obesity.

It is estimated that there are approximately six million morbidly obese persons in the United States alone and that some 60,000 operations are performed annually there in the hope of controlling the condition and its attendant diseases. Hence the need for this book which expresses the anguish, fears, hope and joy of those who have undertaken the journey from the chronic intractable, progressive immolation of morbid obesity towards the long wished-for glorious anonymity of physical normality.

Alex M.C. Macgregor, MD, FACS, FRCSEd
Past President, American Society for Bariatric Surgery

1   The cessation of breathing during sleep

Acknowledgements

Many people deserve my appreciation for their contributions to this endeavor. For those who chose anonymity, accept my grateful nod to your assistance. Dr. Alex Macgregor graciously offered gentle nudges to enhance the accuracy of my information. Dr. Leonard Glade, Dr. Todd Belott and Dr. Patrick Breaux are thanked for their astute observations and opinions regarding real-life cases and the validity of gastric surgery when indicated. Elaine Harrell, with her keen grammatical eye, checked the readability of the chapters.

A special thanks must be given to those marvelous individuals who shared their experiences and gave permission for acknowledgement. Harold Hill, Charles Woodward and Brenda Ingargiola were generous in their honesty and time. Tim Finch skillfully created the surgical descriptive illustrations. Final proofing before submission was done by Joshua Beauchamp and my husband, Keith Parke. Dr. Wilton Beauchamp deserves an 'attaboy' for being an early cheerleader with a frisky red pen. Thanks, too, to Nairda, whose convictions led to my devotion to the project.

Lastly, Amy Lankester-Owen and Jessica Kingsley of Jessica Kingsley Publishers have been supportive and encouraging every step of the way. Words escape.

My sincere indebtedness to each of these and others, who by their preferences or my omission are not mentioned.

Chapter 1
The Problem

Dear Daphne,

Please help me. I am desperate. I have no friends. I hate my job and I'm so tired of people staring at me and making horrible comments about my size. When I eat, I feel better for a little while but afterwards, I just feel worse. I'm 24 years old and weigh 380 pounds. I have tried all kinds of diets and nothing works. What can I do?

Desperate in Denver

Dear Desperate in Denver,

You are describing an addiction disorder. Talk with your physician about options of weight control that you may not have considered. Please contact her immediately. Write and let me know how you are doing. I care.

Daphne

To no one's surprise, obesity looms as a major problem in our society. Twenty-two per cent of the population weighs more than one hundred and twenty per cent of their ideal body weights.[1] This astounding figure translates into an estimated 97 million people.[2] The robust economy and ready availability of food that tastes good combine to create the capacity for overindulgence that many cannot ignore. The prevalence of obesity in our culture has escalated markedly in the last decade.[3] Unless truly motivated, the American adult will ride in his automobile rather than walk and sits in front of the television or computer screen instead of playing ball with her youngsters.

The hour of closing approaches for the bakery. Glenda stands behind the counter, as she has for most of her eight hour shift. Her fatigue borders on exhaustion. Morbidly obese, her job options are few and she is grateful that the bakery manager gave her a chance. She works hard, smiles when she feels like crying and tries to ignore the all-too-frequent remarks made about her weight

On this particular evening, five minutes before closing, a mother with two young boys comes in for croissants. While filling the order, Glenda hears one of the boys remark loudly enough for her to hear, "Bet she eats all the leftovers at the end of the day!"

"Bet this place never has to throw anything away!" the other boy giggles to his brother.

Glenda stares at the two boys, unable to think of a thing to say.

"Wish we didn't have to pay for this stuff. . . we'd be big as cows, too!" The laughing grows louder.

Embarrassed and feeling her face warming, Glenda concentrates on the change she gives the mother.

"Ethan! Where are your manners? Hush, right now!" the mother admonishes. Undeterred, the boy continues to giggle and laugh with his brother as they leave the shop. Their mother glances back apologetically and shrugs her shoulders.

As she counts the money in the drawer and prepares to close for the evening, Glenda feels wounded. She would never think of touching a brownie, a sticky bun or an eclair without paying for them. She slips off her apron scattered with chocolate smudges and cookie crumbs and looks down and then quickly away from the apron she can't take off. She slips a five dollar bill into the cash bag and fills a bakery sack with bearclaws.

With anticipation of the pleasure of sweetness on her tongue and the soothing fullness to come, she clutches her treasure close as she locks the door for the night. Standing on the corner, waiting for the bus, she looks first one direction and then the other. Satisfied that no one is close enough to see her, she gobbles two pastries, one after the other.

Due to the pressures inherent in our culture and the unrealistic societal emphasis toward lean bodies, eating disturbances are on the rise, especially binge eating.[4] Rewards for accomplishments, whether real or imagined, and comfort in times of distress often take the form of special dietary treats.

"Hi, Hal," Glenda greets the familiar bus driver as she pushes herself up the first step of the bus. She tightly clutches the top of the white bag in one dimpled fist.

"Whatchagot in the bag?" the portly Hal leers at the still plump sack of goodies.

For a moment, Glenda thinks to share her bounty but quickly discards the idea. The bearclaws are her treats. "Just some day-olds for breakfast in the morning," she explains as she puffs with the exertion of climbing the four steps.

Hal winks at her. "You never bring me anything."

Glenda glances at the smiling face above three chins as she passes him, "Maybe tomorrow."

The common metabolic disorder, obesity, competes as the most significant public health problem in the United States today.[5] One per cent of those affected, or five million adults, are more than 100 pounds above their ideal body weights and bear the label of severely or morbidly obese.[6] As a toll on society as a whole, the estimated increase in healthcare costs and lost productivity because of the physical effects of the additional weight are $140 billion dollars or seventeen per cent of the total spent on healthcare.[7]

Because of cultural differences in eating habits, economic differences dictating choice in foods and the differences in consideration of obesity in regard to attractiveness, there are twice as many African-American women as Caucasians who meet the criteria of obesity.[8] The incidence in the Hispanic community is one and a half times more frequent than in the Caucasian population.[9]

Thirty minutes later, Glenda shuts the door behind her, grabs a quart of milk from the refrigerator and drops into the big chair in her tiny rented room. Eagerly, compulsively, she consumes the bearclaws. In minutes, the bag emptied, she feels sated and miserable. Pushing herself from the chair with great effort, she pitches the bag and the flattened milk carton into the trash. Sleepy, as she prepares for bed she vows for the thousandth time to start on a diet in the morning.

Efforts, genuine and half-hearted, continue. At any given time, 33–40 per cent of the population of adult females are trying to lose weight. At the same time 20–24 per cent of adult males struggle in the same endeavor. Fully 28 per cent of our population members are just trying to maintain their current weights.[10]

> The following day, Glenda boards the bus again, this time to join her family in Sunday dinner. Italian by heritage, her mother always prepares huge meals, usually spaghetti or lasagna or Glenda's favorite, ravioli. Her mouth waters as she thinks about the flavorful sauces and rich pasta, heavy with cheese and tantalizingly spicy.

The causes for this epidemic, in addition to the availability of food, are genetic and environmental. Our bodies very efficiently promote the storage of fat, especially when supported by a sedentary lifestyle. The tendency for obesity is an inherited legacy. The offspring of obese parents aren't necessarily overweight but the tendency exists in them. Of the genetic/environmental mix, 40–70 per cent of the variation in body mass is inherited.[11]

The morbidly obese may also have a higher incidence of a history of childhood abuse and may exhibit symptoms of post-traumatic stress disorder.[12] Eating to build a wall of fat to insulate themselves effectively prevents others from coming close. By forcing themselves to be unattractive, they subconsciously reject intimate relationships, some of which have caused them pain. Most tragic are those individuals who have such self-loathing that gorging themselves to the point of endangering their lives is a more socially acceptable suicide alternative than use of a pistol or a handful of pills.

Opening the door of the crumbling bungalow of her childhood, Glenda is met with loud greetings from her siblings, the heavenly aromas of simmering marinara sauce and the growl of her father.

"Where the hell you been? Can't you ever be on time for anything? Next time, we start without ya." He is sprawled on the couch, his massive leg, swollen and discolored from poor circulation, is propped unsteadily on the coffee table. A beer can is clutched in one beefy fist. Glenda looks away and mumbles a familiar apology.

A long list of physical ailments plague the morbidly obese. Type II diabetes, a form of diabetes mellitus occuring primarily in adults, strikes with alarming frequency. Hypertension, or high blood pressure, often rears its ugly head, resulting in a proportionate increase in the incidence of strokes. The heart must pump harder to move the blood through the larger mass. A diet high in fat and cholesterol prompts a markedly increased incidence of coronary heart disease. Osteoarthritis, painful and debilitating even for those of slender build, is tragic for the obese person whose affected joints must not only contend with its crippling effects but carry far

more weight with each step than they were designed to
do.

Glenda lumbers into the kitchen.

"Get out of here and go sit down!" her mother
barks. "There's not enough room in here for both of
us!" Easily matching her daughter's girth, the older
woman is finishing the preparations for the meal.
From long habit, Glenda silently obeys her mother
and claims her place at the sturdy dining table.

Diet forgotten, she consumes a huge meal of
spaghetti, Italian bread and homemade cheesecake.
From his place at the head of the table, her father
mocks her gluttony while her mother spoons more
food on her plate.

Incidence of cancer in the morbidly obese exceeds that
of the general population.[13] Colon cancer, breast cancer
and ovarian cancers are specifically more prevalent in
the overweight population.[14] Problems with the identification of suspicious masses in large, fat-laden breasts
make early diagnosis of breast cancer more difficult.
Because of poor self-image and reluctance to disrobe in
front of strangers, morbidly obese women are less likely
to have annual mammograms, which would increase
their chances of stopping the disease in the early stages.

Vocational, academic and medical care opportunities are threatened. Obese workers are perceived as more
slovenly, less dedicated and less able to perform the tasks

assigned and are thus unable to find employment as quickly as their thinner counterparts. A higher lifetime prevalence of anxiety and depression plagues the morbidly obese, bringing challenges not encountered among those of 'normal' size.[15] Beginning in elementary schools, overweight children meet discrimination. Exclusion from activities, taunts from other children and the pervasive sense of being different mark the children emotionally and predispose them to the depression that often surfaces as they age.

> After an afternoon spent watching television and snacking, Glenda leaves her parents' home for the ride to her own sanctuary. She feels depressed and dejected as she wedges her body into the seat of the bus. Why did she eat so much? Was her future just eating and guilt, eating and guilt? A tear slides down her plump cheek as she looks around at the other riders, blessed with smaller bodies.

With reason, because the severely overweight do have numerous medical problems, they feel the discrimination in the field of healthcare. The technical aspects of surgery are more difficult. Control of diseases such as diabetes, heart disease and hypertension is challenging and success rates negatively affected by the depression and denial found in these patients. Their ability to comply with prescription medication and behavioral modification is questioned in the light of the perceived lack of control of their bodies. Well-meaning physicians issue the blithe instruction to 'lose weight or die', not realizing the nearly insurmountable task they have assigned.

Chapter 2
The Candidate

When all other options to provide relief to the unfortunate trapped in a prison of adipose are unavailable, the possibility of surgical intervention may be the answer. Contrary to tabloid hype, 'melting away' of the fat after a surgical procedure involves more than a passive desire to be a healthier size on the part of the patient. A physician, preferably one with a strong bariatric background, can provide a description of the peri-operative experience and explain the complexities of patient obligation.

Not every person afflicted with obesity can stand as a candidate for surgical treatment through alteration of the gastro-intestinal system. The surgery is not a cosmetic one, employed to mold body contours or attain a slim figure so coveted by current society. During the operative procedure, no fat is actually removed from the body. Rather, changing the digestive tract to markedly diminish the desire for food and drastically curb oral intake offers a permanent and irreversible solution to those who have repeatedly and unsuccessfully attempted to trim dangerous amounts of excess weight. These attempts need to be confirmed by documentation.

The ethical bariatric surgeon will consider performing a gastric altering procedure if the candidate carries 100 pounds or more above his or her ideal body weight and has done so for at least five years.[16] Only life-threatening physical conditions caused or made worse by the presence of less than 100 pounds of excess weight will prompt exceptional consideration. Laboratory testing will be done to rule out the presence of glandular diseases such as hypothyroidism (a condition due to deficiency of the thyroid secretion, resulting in lowered basal metabolism) that would indicate a physiological cause for the weight gain. To provide the best chance for success, the candidate will be between 18 and 50 years of age.

Morbid obesity is a chronic, frequently progressive and debilitating disease. Among the systems that can be adversely affected by its presence are skeletal, cardiovascular, gastro-intestinal and auto-immune. Identification of the scope of the problem merits consideration of the surgical alternative when no other method of weight control is effective.

In the public's viewpoint, the misconception persists that excess body weight is determined by acquired food habits and uncontrolled desire or lack of willpower. The expectation that morbidly obese individuals can overcome inherited tendencies in order to be thin is a fantasy. Cultural and environmental stressors that provoke binge eating are ingrained and can be nearly impossible to overcome. Psychological barriers and socioeconomic circumstances each contribute, in part, to the often hopeless condition of these people.

Identified scientifically, specific proteins are manufactured by fat cells that have been proven to be, in part, the determinant of appetite. The role of these substances is to control feelings of satiety, or fullness. As much a part of a person's physical make-up as blue eyes or brown skin, the characteristics of these proteins have been established at conception. Their regulatory functions in a morbidly obese individual are inadequate to provide a barrier to indiscriminate excess.

Binge eating, identified as a frequent practice in the obese population[17], escalates during times of stress. The level of stress necessary to spur an episode of gluttonous intake varies as does the time frame to cessation. Food as a reward or as a comfort only provides eventual guilt and additional stress.

From a childhood all too often marked by mockery, forced deprivation of food and even emotional or sexual abuse, the morbidly obese adult is left psychologically fragile. Deep depression, classically described as anger turned inward, and its partner, anxiety, cripple them. In fact making the problem worse, the response to these onslaughts is food. The enormous effort required to adhere to a dietary denial program cannot be found in a delicate psyche trying to cope with daily guilt and ridicule.

Diets high in carbohydrates and fats predispose to excess weight. Whether cultural or economic in origin, a constant intake of fried foods, rich gravies, and unlimited amounts of sweets to the exclusion of fruits, vegetables and lean meats condemns those already prone to bearing excess weight to outright obesity. With admitted exceptions, the chosen foods are those to which the person is accustomed, the foods that were offered during childhood. In some cultures, robust appetites and buxom figures are taken to indicate a measure of good health, power or well-being and as such, excessive intake is encouraged. Large women can be perceived as attractive by men and thus influenced to carry dangerously massive weights.

Periodic loss of weight and subsequent regaining of that weight causes additional stress on a body struggling for balance. As the cycle continues with the addition of yet more weight with each rotation the choice of options narrows and recourse to operative intervention becomes more likely. The emotional toll of these cycles builds with each failed attempt, leaving guilt and further erosion of self-image.

If methods such as counseling, conventional dieting and exercise fail, surgical treatment may become the only effective method of achieving long-term weight control for those whose lives are endangered by obesity. Risks abound for those undergoing gastric surgery, in part because of the enormous amounts of fat tissue present. Visualization of the targeted surgical area is impaired by a wall of fat, often greater than six inches in depth. Inadvertent excision of tissues and/or inaccurate or inadequate suturing occurs for that reason. Respiratory integrity during and following the procedure is often compromised because of the extensive amount of chest corpulence, requiring artificial ventilation. Despite these and other risks, surgical treatment may be the only recourse to sustain life.

The person contemplating gastric surgery for severe obesity must be realistic, committed and informed. Expectations of a magical cure at the hands of another are misplaced. A focused and dedicated investment must be made by the patient himself for the results to be optimal.

The prospective surgical candidate should not expect to attain his ideal body weight through surgical intervention alone. After surgery the amount of weight loss is variable and unpredictable. Loss is projected to be a half to two thirds of the excess weight[18]. Weight is predicted to stabilize slightly above ideal body weight. Depending on his or her original weight, the choice of the procedure performed and the commitment of the patient, the results achieved will vary. Importantly, even small amounts of sacrificed weight yield impressive health benefits.

The commitment made by the patient must be one to last a lifetime. In addition to medical pre-operative clearance, regular and frequent visits to a physician experienced in obesity management must be rigorously self-enforced after the procedure. Recognition of the early signs of complications means they can be identified and treated immediately, avoiding life-threatening problems. The choice of a physician is a critical one and bears careful investigation before establishing a professional relationship.

Equally crucial is the recognition that a total change in dietary habits must be made. Not only will the quantity of food eaten need to be markedly reduced, but the nutritional value of the food will have to be analyzed for vitamin and mineral content, consistency, texture and digestability suitable for the individual. With attention to patient preferences, a subsistence program will be established after surgery and continuously evaluated for patient tolerance. Preparation, monitoring and support for changes in diet will be provided by a member of the bariatric medicine team, most frequently a dietician or nutritionist. As the patient's tastes adapt and his or her body adjusts to the changes, dietary shifts will be necessary and encouraged.

Depending on the specific surgery performed, a regimen of vitamin therapy may be needed indefinitely. From results of blood tests and observation for evidence of physical changes in the hair, teeth, nails and skin, the physicians following the patient are best able to ascertain which nutrients need to be added. Vitamin C, B12 and iron supplements are the most frequently required.

The essential element that is the patient's willpower can't be ignored. After surgery, high calorie liquids, ice creams, puddings and other treats can be tolerated in small amounts, resulting in low weight loss. The patient must recognize that the small amounts of food allowed by the reduced capacity of the stomach must be carefully selected. In order to avoid unpleasant side-effects as well as painful ones, following the prescribed diet is compulsory.

An exercise plan is strongly advocated in conjunction with the surgical therapy. As the weight vanishes, exercise will become easier. Regular walking not only aids in accelerating the metabolism but firms tissues as the fat disappears. Another member of the support team, a physical therapist or exercise specialist, will provide guidelines to tailor a patient-specific program.

The need for psychological counseling cannot be overstated. With the high incidence of depression and anxiety seen in the morbidly obese, other problems can be masked to the untrained observer. In order to evaluate the level of success possible after surgery, a profile should be undertaken by a trained mental health professional. Adapting to radical alteration in body image, changes in self-nurturing techniques and other shifts in lifestyle will require expert consultation. The degree of motivation of the potential surgical candidate can also be gauged by a competent professional prior to the operation. Psychological analysis thus provides a tool for predicting the outcome of the entire peri-operative procedure unavailable through other avenues.

An alternative focus must be established to replace eating in the post-surgical patient. Prior to surgery, the amount of food and number of calories required to achieve and maintain weights in excess of 100 pounds over ideal body weight demand a great deal of expense, time and effort. Ideally, replacement options should be in place prior to the surgical procedure. At the very least, choices of alternative recreation should be considered. Initially, such activities as reading, playing cards or attending a class of interest might be preferential. Ultimately, more arduous physical endeavors such as mall walking or bicycle riding will be possible. Patients' interests are as individual as the owner. Each must determine his or her own activities and diversions as part of the ongoing commitment to success.

The importance of a support system in place through the entire weight loss experience cannot be exaggerated. Consultation with family members should include an exploration of behaviors, both negative and positive, that will impact on the patient's chance for success. Comprehensive information and instructions given to the family as well as to the patient, in a deliberately non-judgmental manner, establish a good relationship with the team members and foster future communication. Much of the material provided may be forgotten and reinforcement will be necessary. The aforementioned psychological counselor will suggest a support approach distinctive to the individual. Ongoing accessibility of that professional for the family to answer questions and offer assistance gives the patient one more advantage in winning the most crucial battle of his or her life.

The decision to undergo radical gastric surgery to alter intake is one that should be made in partnership with all members of the healthcare team. The surgeon, medical doctor, dietician, physical therapist and psychologist or social worker each bring invaluable expertise and knowledge.

The complications that can occur should be discussed fully prior to making the operative decision. The patient must be included in formulation of the plan of care. Only an individual who feels fully prepared is equal to the commitment required to make the experience a success.

Chapter 3
The Surgery

The two surgical procedures most frequently performed by bariatric specialists are the vertical banded gastroplasty and variations of the gastric bypass. Research regarding modifications of each of the operations is ongoing in an attempt to achieve the goals of maximum weight loss with minimal side-effects and few complications.

First introduced in 1982 in the United States, the vertical banded gastroplasty (VBG) markedly reduces the size of the functioning portion of the stomach. Appetite and the limit of the amount of food ingested are decreased, thus forcing a reduction in calories consumed and subsequent weight loss.

In VBG, the restrictive gastric pouch is created by stapling the stomach walls together and fashioning a window to allow placement of the Marlex mesh collar around the outlet of the pouch (see Figure 1).

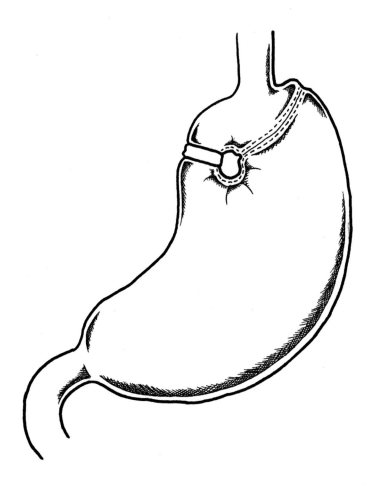

Figure 1: Vertical Banded Gastroplasty

The circumference of the band is calibrated to attain a diameter of approximately one centimeter, comparable to the size of a little finger. A vertical staple line, leading away from the window and terminating near the juncture of the stomach and esophagus, completes the pouch. After different locations were tested, placement of the pouch in the inner curvature of the stomach was proven to be most effective for successful weight loss because the increase in muscular density of this area hinders stretching.

Optimum results from the procedure have been correlated to a pouch initially holding fourteen milliliters of fluid, approximately three teaspoonsful. Because of the minuscule capacity, rapid filling with satiation is attained. The band prevents immediate emptying and a sense of satisfaction is retained for a longer period of time.

Short hospital stays, estimated at one to two days[19], and rapid recovery times are but two of the many advantages of VBG over the more complex gastric bypass procedure. A purely restrictive process, VBG does not disrupt the normal digestive process, and avoids the complication of anemia. The number of post-operative complications seen with VBG is fewer than with the gastric bypass.

Tolerance for sweets is unaffected by the anatomic restriction enforced by VBG. Soft drinks, ice cream, puddings and other fat-laden liquids or semi-liquids pass rapidly through the pouch. For that reason, bariatric professionals do not recommend VBG for those patients who are sweet-eaters, citing weight-loss failure and frequent need for further, more extensive operations to achieve the goal of reduced intake. From the research obtained from successful outcomes achieved to date, professionals performing the procedure recommend its being done on patients whose excess weight is not more than one hundred pounds.

Despite positioning to prevent such an occurrence, stretching of the tiny pouch can be effected with repeated episodes of excessive intake. Initially, vomiting and discomfort will develop with over-eating but these lessen as the pouch enlarges. Much lower weight loss than is possible with compliance in the patient is recorded as a result of the increase in intake. For those morbidly obese individuals whose health is adversely affected by their weights, surgical re-entry into the abdominal cavity to carry out more extensively restrictive procedures proves necessary.

Peak weight loss is obtained usually within 18 to 24 months post-operatively[20] but maintenance of weight loss is shorter in duration with VBG than gastric bypass. Positive initial success is frequently reversed in the years following surgery as the pouch enlarges.

Change in the actual method of intake will be necessary for patient comfort. Eating slowly is mandatory as is thorough chewing of each mouthful of food. The small outlet of the pouch requires partial oral digestion of the food before it will pass through easily. Vomiting results if the technique is not followed and large pieces of foodstuff are swallowed. Successful practice of this procedure must be monitored post-operatively, especially during the first three months, to circumvent protein and/or vitamin deficiencies.

The permanence of a vertical banding procedure must be considered by the potential candidate. Once the integrity of the stomach has been interrupted, no surgical procedure has been proven effective in converting its function and stability to its pre-operative state. If the surgery is unsuccessful, or if complications arise, further operative procedures are longer in terms of anesthesia, require a higher level of physician expertise due to technical obstacles and harbor a greater potential for eventual difficulties.

Mechanical complications are listed among the most frequently observed problems seen post-operatively1. Erosion of the Martex band into the stomach tissue can cause ulcers internally as well as immediately under the band. Disruption of part or all of the staple line has also been documented, resulting in intake routeing to the main portion of the stomach and a total absence of weight loss. The potential for disruption of the staple line is increased when greater amounts of food are consumed than are recommended.

Infection looms as a possibility in any invasive procedure. In VBG, leakage of gastric fluid through the staple line of the stomach can be responsible for failure of the internal area to heal or more serious, peritonitis. The entry wound through the skin is a potential site for infection and cleansing of the area must be carried out diligently as instructed by the physician to avoid contamination. The dangers inherent in surgery are particularly hazardous to the morbidly obese individual. Deep venous thrombosis can result from even a short period of inactivity due to the chronic stress on the vessels. Unpleasant but treatable as an isolated occurrence, the presence of a blood clot in an extremity can be potentially deadly if the clot breaks loose and travels to the lungs or the heart. Since bariatric surgery is often performed as an adjunct therapy for physical problems, those difficulties can be magnified during and immediately after the procedure. Blood pressure, liver function and pulmonary function must be evaluated pre-operatively and monitored closely in the hours after major surgery. The importance of a complete physical examination, including blood tests and x-rays before hospitalization, cannot be stressed too strongly as part of the preparation for surgery.

Because of the increased bulk of the chest tissue, greatly obese individuals often find sleeping in a sitting position more comfortable than lying down. The lungs, like balloons, inflate more easily when the pressure is minimized. Unfortunately, the position necessary for surgery is flat and post-operative mechanical ventilation is occasionally necessary for proper lung expansion. The length of time for which artificial intervention is needed depends on the patient's overall state of health, the length of the surgical procedure and response to anesthesia. Another factor predisposing to lung problems is limited lung expansion brought on by the pain in the incisional area associated with deep breathing.

With evidence of higher weight losses that are maintained for a longer period of time, physicians frequently recommend a gastric bypass to those patients whose weight is in excess of the ideal by 125 pounds or more, snack constantly, crave junk food or never feel full. Combining the creation of a small stomach pouch with a shortening and re-routeing of the small intestine, the goals of limited intake and decreased absorption of calories and nutrients are achieved.

In the gastric bypass procedure, the portion of the stomach that will not be used is literally separated from the pouch. Instead of utilizing staples to delineate the two compartments, a gastric transection is performed. By dividing the staple line and oversewing the cut ends, a more permanent and stable division is secured. Originally developed by Dr. Edward E. Mason of the University of Iowa, the operation constructs a one ounce pouch with a limb of intestine attached. The body of the stomach is left intact to preserve nerves in the area and

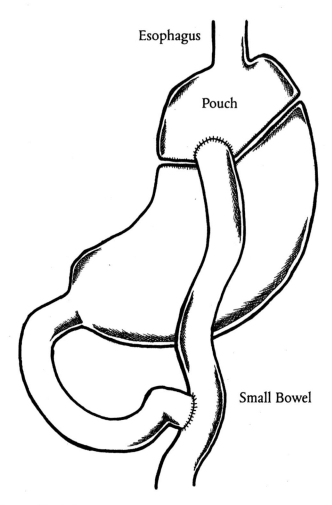

Figure 2: Gastric Bypass

carefully fixed in the abdomen to avoid torsion, or twisting, at the outlet which is attached at a lower point in the small intestine. The term 'Roux en Y' was given the limb configuration because of the y-shaped appearance of the pouch-intestinal joining (See Figure 2).

Requiring a minimum of three days hospitalization, gastric bypass is a more lengthy and complicated procedure than the VBG but practitioners boast proven higher weight losses. Significant weight loss is always achieved with two-thirds of the excess weight being a reasonable expectation[21]. Gastric bypass has facilitated a loss of at least half of the excess weight in 80 per cent of those having the surgery[22].

The length of time that liquids and puréed foods are recommended after gastric bypass is longer than with a VBG because of the complexity of the surgery. Up to four weeks with no solid food allows the transected stomach to heal properly and disruption is avoided. Because of the larger outlet of the stomach, as compared to that of the VBG, meat and chicken will be tolerated after a period of adjustment. From the beginning of the post-operative period, the demand of the body for nutritional supplements exists. Vitamin B12 and Calcium are absorbed from the digested food by the portion of the small intestine that is bypassed by the surgery. For this reason, those specific additives as well as a multi-vitamin must be included in the permanent dietary regimen.

The immediate post-operative risks include pulmonary embolus (blood clot to the lung) which is the most common cause, although rare, of early post-operative death. With a 0.16–1 per cent occurrence, depending on the reporting source, the second most commonly seen serious complication is a leak at the juncture where the small intestine has been secured to the pouch[23]. Gastric dilatation of the newly formed reservoir also has been known to occur, due to an obstruction or simply spontaneously. Relief of that condition requires an endoscopic procedure to identify and remove the cause and alleviate the symptoms of discomfort.

The most publicized complication, which can occur as an early or late event, is the 'dumping syndrome'. A side-effect of the actual surgery, the symptoms of the syndrome are triggered by the intake of refined sugar by the patient. These include rapid heart beat, nausea, tremors and a faint feeling with occasional accompanying diarrhea. Episodes of dumping syndrome quickly discourage the patient from sneaking forbidden sweets. No correlation has been made between dumping and increased weight loss.

Another complication seen after the patient has stabilized from the surgery is a narrowing of the tissue where the intestine meets the pouch. Essentially, this arises from scar tissue development. A balloon inflation performed through endoscopy easily relieves the stricture. Other late complications are most commonly results of nutrient deficiency. These include frank anemia from iron deficiency and osteoporosis from calcium deficiency. Particular attention must be paid to post-menopausal women for early evidence of osteoporosis. Being at risk prior to surgery, these women are especially prone to its incidence.

A three to ten per cent occurrence of ulcers at the site of the intestinal-pouch junction has been reported[24]. Medically treatable, this condition is readily reversed when recognized early in its development.

An overall 30 day post-procedural complication rate approaching 7 per cent is reported by the International Bariatric Surgery Registry[25]. Patient compliance measures aren't factored into this figure and the percentage would surely plunge with their inclusion. Considering the 0.17 per cent death rate attributed to the effects of gastric surgery [26], inclusive of both VBG and gastric bypass, the serious complication rate is low. Judging from the number of medical problems existent in the population of patients, the safety of the procedures exceeds expectation.

Chapter 4

John

John slowly shook his head back and forth, a shock of unruly graying blond hair falling over his forehead. "I had control, with God's help, over every part of my life but the eating. The devil was firmly in control of that department."

A minister by vocation and calling, John was known for his compassion and warmth. A popular leader, he humbly and energetically prepared weekly sermons, provided comfort for the sick and dying, performed weddings and acted as administrator of the church day care. Neither a drinker nor a smoker, he asked God for help in rejecting temptations and tried to rely on His support. He prayed fervently for the strength to turn his back on second and third helpings at meal times. John just didn't feel God was lifting him away from the vice of overeating. He felt adrift and powerless.

"I'm a passionate preacher. Five minutes into a sermon, sweat would be running down my face. Sometimes, I'd have to cut short the sermon because I couldn't catch my breath from the pacing and the shouting.

"I knew that this…this obsession with food was my cross to bear. I begged and pleaded for God to intervene and He didn't. My faith was challenged and I began to doubt." His voice rose and just as quickly dropped again.

"Then…the answer came. I'll never know who tipped him off but a fine Christian doctor, a surgeon, called the church office and asked to speak to me. After chatting a short while, he explained he did stomach surgeries so fat folks would be forced to eat less. Then he asked me if I would be interested."

John had answered reluctantly: "I'm interested but I don't have that kind of money, Doctor. I'm a poor preacher,"

"Let me worry about the fees," the doctor told John and promised to call the following day for an answer.

John hurriedly left the church and went home to talk to Marie. "I have doubts," he admitted. "To alter my God-given body just doesn't seem right."

After listening carefully and asking a few questions, Marie offered her opinion. "John, God sent this man to you. He gave him the skill to heal and to help. Don't turn your back on this chance."

Marie was right as usual. John continued his story. "I knew I had a lot of God's work to do and I didn't have much time left to do it, the way I was feeling." He was experiencing difficulty with breathing and pains in his ankles and knees and had a genuine fear of a stroke from high blood pressure, unchecked by a variety of medications.

"So, we did it!" He described committing to a decision finalized only after lengthy episodes of prayer and meditation.

"Half of the membership of the church turned out the day of the operation," he mentioned with some pride.

"The other half would have been there but they were working to support the first half!" His hearty laugh boomed.

"Flowers everywhere, but no food. No food was allowed."

John rode a stretcher to the operating room with Marie at his side until she was left behind at the swinging doors. "The prayer chain started when I left my room. Each person had ten minutes then passed on to someone else. I wasn't afraid. . .how could I be?"

John has tasted a lot of dishes at church suppers since that fateful day. He has lost two hundred and thirty pounds. He takes no medication and walks two miles a day. A regular attendee, he frequently addresses the group meetings of the bariatric support group. When asked to do so, he accompanies others to the hospital as a show of support.

Leaning forward and gesturing heavenward with a pointed finger, John expressed a final thought. "Yes, God answers prayer but in His time, not ours."

Chapter 5
Viola

Viola rolled from her desk to the "outbox" of the Judson Memorial Hospital Social Services office with a completed psycho-social evaluation in hand. The wheels of her chair, the third in as many years and purchased specifically for her, groaned with the effort. Upholstery on the front of the seat cushion had succumbed to the incessant rubbing of Viola's thighs, tufts of soft yellow matting bursting from the rupture. None of the other social workers considered using the chair for fear of a sharp rebuke from Viola.

Even the short trip caused Viola's breathing to escalate and beads of perspiration to sprinkle her forehead. Remembering a group meeting scheduled on the Psych unit, she shoved herself from the chair, lifting a bulk equivalent to two additional bodies. As she did so, the bottom drawer of a file cabinet slid free and she struck her knee sharply on its edge. The flash of pain brought a wave of nausea and paralyzed the leg. Viola fell against the nearest desk, gasping. Turning on her uninjured leg, she fell into her chair, nearly toppling as she fought for balance.

Moments later, the door to the office opened and another of the social workers entered the room. Finding Viola grimacing and massaging her knee, her usual ruddy complexion sheened with gray and the file cabinet drawer gaping at her side, he immediately realized what had happened.

Long minutes later, Viola was being wheeled to the Emergency Department in a "big boy" wheelchair by a hefty orderly, headed toward the first of a series of medical encounters that would lead to a new life.

None of her co-workers could remember seeing Viola eat during her six years at Judson. Even at hospital parties, if she attended at all, she would sip a glass of diet cola. A long commute from her home provided a good excuse to avoid most such social gatherings and peoples' silent stares. Private and often uncommunicative, she had erected an emotional wall that few attempted to scale.

Reared the youngest of five and the only daughter, Viola initially related a storybook childhood to her counselor in the mandatory sessions prior to gastric surgery. Only after intensive probing did she admit that her mother had evicted her father from their middle-class existence when she was only eight years of age. Vague and evasive, she alluded to a discovery made by her mother that fractured their family. Her father had been caught sexually abusing his youngest child. Viola steadfastly refused to elaborate and despite her intellectual abilities and education, denied the impact of the events on her life as an adult.

Shortly after her father's departure, Viola the child began to gain weight. Always a hearty eater, she welcomed the treats and extra helpings encouraged by her mother and grandmother. Anxious to assuage their own senses of guilt, the women offered the only comfort that Viola seemed to accept and enjoy.

High school graduation pictures show a markedly obese young woman. With doe-like eyes and plump cheeks, a serious Viola stared defensively from the pages of the yearbook. At 342 pounds, she knew her future depended on academic performance. During the ceremony marking her class' passage, Viola received accolades as the salutatorian, second in scholarship in her class of 200. She had never had a date, never attended a football game and could name only a scant few of her classmates considered as acquaintances and none as close friends. The pattern of her life had been established before she entered college to fulfill a lifelong dream. She wanted to be a social worker.

Attending a local junior college whose admission policy was open and living at home with her solicitous mother, Viola rapidly distinguished herself academically. Traveling to class in a sturdy truck purchased for her by proud older brothers, she never missed a class nor an assignment. Graduation from junior college and admission to the state university, courtesy of a 4.0 gradepoint average, found Viola weighing 375 pounds. The cab of her precious truck was full of discarded greasy donut bags, empty fried chicken boxes and Snicker wrappers.

Graduation from the university brought no job offers despite Viola's stellar academic credentials. She experienced no difficulty getting interviews but none of the prospective employers followed with offers. Since she was intent on staying near the security of her mother, Viola's opportunities were further diminished. Clad in outfits fashioned by her grandmother, Viola faced cool receptions and the familiar stares.

After months of discouraging failure to find a job in the field of her choice, Viola had accepted that she might never achieve her goal of working in social service. A sales position at a fabric store occupied her time and provided spending money. When her mother excitedly called the store one afternoon to tell her about an advertisement in the classified section of the paper requesting applications for the position of social worker at Judson Memorial Hospital, Viola was skeptical but hopeful. Ninety minutes from her home, Judson enjoyed a reputation for its liberal hiring practices and offered the opportunity to work in a modern, progressive environment. Reluctant at the thought of further rejection, Viola half-heartedly agreed to inquire at the hospital.

Much to her surprise, the first interview with Human Resources went well and she was invited back for a second. Giddy with anticipation, Viola accepted an entry level social worker's position as offered. Hoping to seize the moment to change the behaviors of her life, she vowed to make a serious effort at dietary control. Successful and insightful in other areas of her life, she once again met with defeat when trying to limit her food intake. Secretive to the point of being aloof, Viola shared her intent with none of her new co-workers, members of a willing and trained support system. They couldn't provide help if she didn't ask.

In the six years prior to her accident, Viola rarely missed work and carried her caseload successfully. Due to her escalating weight, she encountered increasing difficulties in maneuvering from one unit to another but never shirked her duties. Regular pay increases allowed the purchase of the home next door to her mother and the eventual replacement of her truck. She was abstemious by day, but her evenings were spent gorging and her weight soared to over 450 pounds. She recognized her need for help intellectually, but dealt with her psychological and physical disabilities by denying any problems adamantly. Injury of her knee prompted a time of unwelcome self-examination and a reluctant decision to act if her career and dreams were to be salvaged.

After emergency treatment at Judson, Viola returned home and met with her private physician. In the weeks following, enforced rest and self-treatment with anti-inflammatory medications failed to restore the ability of the joint to bear weight and she endured a series of consultations with orthopedic surgeons. None would consider operating on the offending knee, citing the probability of surgical disappointment and the high possibility of surgical or anesthetic complication. Each and every physician encouraged Viola to lose at least 150 pounds before surgery could be considered. Continuing to deny the obvious, she sat at home, eating. Her bills were paid, courtesy of workman's compensation. Denial manifest itself in her certainty that she would walk again if the injury was given enough time to heal.

Her decision to submit to a gastric bypass was prompted by financial worries, not by an admission that it was physically necessary. The Workman's Compensation Board had revoked her payments, indicating the time period for recuperation of the knee had expired, and she was forced to subsist on long-term disability payments. In order to maintain ownership of her house and meet her other financial obligations, Viola accepted that she had to get back to work. After three canceled appointments, she met with a bariatric surgeon, referred by her primary physician. Skilled in evading emotional issues, Viola nonetheless received a positive evaluation from the psychologist on the team. In spite of her refusal to attend preparatory group meetings, ostensibly due to her inability to ambulate, a gastric bypass was performed, Viola's family at her side.

The first weeks of recovery were remarkable for the miserable nausea and vomiting Viola endured. She stayed in bed, attended by her mother. Each teaspoon of liquid seemed to trigger waves of illness and heat. Fighting to retain the soups and purées prepared by her mother, she daily regretted her decision to have the surgery. Her knee still ached and she clung to a walker when forced to leave her bed.

Four months after surgery, Viola had lost seventeen pounds. She limped in to see her doctor, only to be angrily told that she wasn't making an effort on her own behalf. The doctor quizzed her mother about the foods she was preparing for Viola and discovered she was supplying high calorie cream soups and sauces for the softened vegetables and gravies for the mashed potatoes. Her mother insisted Viola preferred those tasty additions and grumpily maintained that her daughter required "good food" to get well. Viola silently listened to the exchange. When the doctor questioned her lack of activity, she finally responded. She couldn't exercise, her knee prevented any activity. She couldn't drive and she hesitated to inconvenience her family by asking any of them to take her to group therapy. She steadfastly denied the necessity for psychological support. Her excuses were colorful and her stubbornness well entrenched.

Only when the physician threatened her with withdrawal of treatment did she agree to embrace the program and seriously promise to follow the suggested regimen. Her mother met with dieticians. Her brothers willingly rotated the chore of delivering Viola to regular group therapy meetings. With attendance in a water exercise class three times a week, she finally began to lose weight.

Having been told of Viola's surgery by the employee handling insurance coverage at the hospital, her co-workers occasionally called to wish her well. She never admitted to having undergone gastric surgery; instead asserted that she was going through rehabilitation for her knee injury. The calls became less frequent. After a year, the hospital dropped her from its employment rolls, promising her a job if one was open when she was ready to return.

Eighteen months after leaving Judson, Viola came back to her old job, 150 pounds lighter. She was walking, although awkwardly, and her self-esteem had soared. In response to delighted observations of all who saw her in her new clothes, she praised the merits of exercise and physical rehabilitation but denied any gastric surgical intervention. To admit to having a bypass was to admit defeat and weakness. For Viola, those traits were unacceptable.

Chapter 6
Jerry Michael

Jerry Michael discovered cigarettes when he was twelve years old. His best friend, Brian, told him that his mother stayed slim by smoking rather than eating. Already hefty and the brunt of peer jokes, he leapt at the chance to curb his monstrous appetite. The first few cigarettes were repulsive but with practice, he became a tolerant smoker and by the age of thirteen, was fully addicted to the demands of a pack a day habit. By that time, he had discarded the original motivation for his smoking and simply coupled the two addictions.

Jerry Michael's parents objected to his indulgence but tolerated it, thinking it was a fad. Years of watching their only child ostracized because of his size led them to overlook protectively his few shortcomings.

Jerry Michael detected no change in his appetite or his size when he started smoking. In spite of his increasing addiction to nicotine, he continued the mammoth breakfasts, lunches consisting of Twinkie six packs or double root beer floats and suppers of meat, potatoes, bread and dessert (with extra helpings). School breaks involved trips to the back of the building where Jerry Michael sucked a couple of smokes with his addicted classmates, then made a stop at the junk food machine for a sugar fix before arriving, usually late, to his next class.

According to his parents, Jerry Michael was popular with his classmates. Every Friday night football or basketball game found him in a crowd of teenagers, urging its team to victory. Until his size prohibited such activities, he was involved in weekend car washes to raise money for school projects, miniature golf with his favorite friends or mall cruising on Saturdays. He became a familiar sight in the streets of his small town, driving his vintage Volvo, usually filled with raucous boys looking for a good time.

Colds and attacks of influenza began to plague Jerry Michael. By his third year in high school, he could only sleep when he was propped up with four pillows to aid his breathing. Particularly susceptible to respiratory infections because of the additional load of his weight and the side-effects of smoking, his lungs struggled. Illness became more frequent and more severe with each occurrence.

When he was seventeen, Jerry Michael was unable to shake a persistent cough and fever and was admitted to a local hospital diagnosed with pneumonia. The weather had been unusually erratic and the infection followed a long stretch of smoke breaks in the freezing drizzle outside and returns to the overheated classrooms. He was released after five days with stern admonitions from his physician and a course of antibiotics and respiratory treatments. His doctor told him the smoking had to stop and at least some of the weight had to be lost. Jerry Michael weighed 433 pounds.

In the months that followed, he truly made an effort. He joined a local support group for those who wished to lose excess weight and miserably cut his intake.

Although difficult, shedding pounds was easy relative to stopping smoking. Nicotine gum, nicotine patches, support groups and hypnosis all failed to dull Jerry Michael's desire to smoke. Jerry Michael's father related one time when, smelling smoke, he went to his son's room to scold him. On opening the door, he found his child with a cigarette in his hand and tears streaming down his face. Instead of chastising him, he held his son and cried with him.

During his senior year in high school, Jerry Michael's father died from a heart attack. Devastated by her loss, his mother gave up her efforts at supporting Jerry Michael's dieting. Left to his own devices and grieving himself, he returned to food for comfort. The weight he had lost quickly returned.

Completion of high school brought Jerry Michael to the local vo-tech college. He registered for various classes in an effort to find an area of interest. Although intelligent, diligent and personable, he was forced to drop out of school during the second semester due to his frequent absences. Upper respiratory infections always heralded full blown pneumonia and hospitalizations became routine. An oxygen tank had been installed in his bedroom, and he always had to keep an inhaler with him.

Ventilator support became necessary to allow clearance of tenacious secretions during one of his later admissions to the hospital. With a tube inserted in his trachea and a machine dictating the timing, depth and oxygen content of each breath, Jerry Michael struggled against the restraints that prevented him from dislodging the tube. He required massive amounts of sedation to remain quiet and was placed on a special, large bed to accommodate his size and allow him to be turned. After weaning from the machine, weeks of antibiotic therapy, respiratory treatments and cessation from nicotine, he was allowed to return home. Before his discharge, his physician approached him and his mother with an urgent suggestion. That Jerry Michael consider a gastric bypass.

Initially, both the patient and his mother felt that this drastic measure was out of the question. Assurances that he would otherwise have to continue to return to the horrors of the ventilator eventually compelled them to consider the surgery and they agreed to meet with the bariatric surgeon recommended by the lung specialist.

Reluctance turned to enthusiasm after meeting with the surgeon. She described the procedure, related the preparations and most important to Jerry Michael, showed him before and after pictures of morbidly obese patients who had successfully undergone the surgery. He was further buoyed after attending a group meeting of those individuals who offered support and encouragement.

Jerry Michael entered the hospital to have the gastric bypass weighing 502 pounds. He was advised that ventilatory management would be necessary following the operation and accepted its inevitability.

His mother met with the hospital dieticians for guidance in the preparation of his meals. She arranged for appointments with Jerry Michael's psychologist for counsel. She spent the day of the operation, in the waiting room of the surgery at the hospital.

Surgery was successful. Because of the necessity of the ventilator, Jerry Michael was moved to the Intensive Care Unit of the hospital. Not surprisingly, he didn't require as much sedation as during his previous bout with pneumonia and restraints weren't necessary. He was working with, instead of against, the nursing staff.

Weaning from the ventilator progressed more slowly than the physicians had anticipated. Jerry Michael acquired a particularly virulent form of infection and his lungs didn't respond to medication or treatments. Various consultants were contacted and numerous antibiotics and therapies were attempted. Although frequently febrile and sedated for comfort, the patient was advised of the activities surrounding his care. He did his best to maintain a positive attitude and help the nurses. His mother was in constant attendance.

Shortly after midnight on the fifteenth day after surgery, Jerry Michael started to struggle against the ventilator. He was agitated and anxious. His color had turned to a dusky gray and the monitor recorded the oxygen saturation in his blood was 70 per cent, down from a previous 98 per cent. Nurses frantically called the physicians and increased the amount of oxygen being delivered from the machine. Suspecting a mucous plug in his airway, they irrigated and suctioned the tracheal tube. There was no positive response. The oxygen level in his blood continued to drop and he lost consciousness. Life-saving drugs were given to no avail. Resuscitative measures failed. Jerry Michael died at 22.

An autopsy performed the following day revealed a massive pulmonary embolus – a blood clot lodged in the main artery of the lung which prevented oxygen-rich blood from being delivered to the body. In order to avoid one of the most common complications for the morbidly obese undergoing surgery, preventive measures had been exercised. Support stockings were in use as were compression devices on Jerry Michael's legs. Infusions of medication to thin the blood were continuous. The nicotine abuse and morbid obesity had created a perfect environment for the development of the embolus.

Jerry Michael's mother clutched the framed graduation picture of her son to her breast as she rocked back and forth.

Chapter 7

Virginia

Virginia remembers vividly the day she stepped from a Greyhound bus into the streets of a sleepy Nebraska town and a new life. She was sixteen years of age and heavy with her first pregnancy. She had traded the boredom of high school classes, the bedroom shared with two younger sisters, Sundays at church pre-occupied with her daydreams and an admittedly shift-less boyfriend four years her senior for the freedom and drudgery of independence.

Virginia quickly landed a job. Because of her cheerful personality, ready laughter, and despite her obvious physical condition, the owner of a local diner offered her a chance to earn her own way. Generous tips provided money and Virginia lovingly furnished her rented room ready for the expected child.

The novelty of delivering heaping platefuls of crispy fried chicken with the trimmings or immense chunks of saucy meatloaf to truckers and tourists lost its appeal as her bulk increased. In order to combat her growing fatigue, Virginia fortified herself with doses of caffeine in the form of full-strength Pepsi. Additional pounds piled on her already chubby frame, not all the results of pregnancy. When Virginia entered the county hospital to deliver Bart, she weighed 190 pounds. Expecting a huge weight change after the birth of her son, she was disappointed with a 14 pounds difference when she returned to work at the diner.

Understanding and concerned over the plight of the new mother, Virginia's boss allowed her to bring her baby to work with her on the midnight shift. Good waitresses were difficult to find and Virginia worked hard. Bart spent his first years of life sleeping in the boss' office. His mother grabbed naps with her baby during the day.

Intent on bettering herself, Virginia studied for and passed the GED. When Bart was only a toddler, she enrolled in a junior college nearby. Co-workers volunteered to watch the child while she attended classes. All the while, she persisted in her weight gain. High calorie soft drinks and diner food still allowed her to stay awake on her night shifts and support herself and Bart.

Not long after Bart's birth, she met Lee, who had been hired to replace the night cook. A master of the grill, Lee prepared food with enthusiasm and skill and the few night customers steadily grew in number. As the months went by, he and Virginia became good friends. He particularly liked Bart and would spend time with the little boy whenever he could. He spoiled them both, preparing special dishes for Virginia and watching Bart when she studied for finals. He seemed to take delight in providing them with surprises such as trips to the circus or a nearby traveling carnival. To Virginia's relief, he never mentioned her size and ignored others when they made comments.

Over the protests of her co-workers and friends, she nurtured the progress of the relationship, hoping for marriage. Because of his effeminate mannerisms and extreme privacy about his past, many suspected Lee was gay. Virginia only recognized that he was good to her, good to Bart and willing to overlook her shortcomings.

They were married two days after she completed her studies to become an Emergency Medical Technician III, a paramedic. Having packed the battered station wagon with their few belongings and one boisterous child, the newlyweds waved goodbyes and departed for the big city where Virginia had secured employment. Lee resigned his job at the diner and never worked again.

At first, Lee maintained he couldn't find work. He stayed in their modest apartment with Bart and always had a big meal ready when Virginia returned from duty.

Bobby was born ten months after their marriage and Lee shouldered the care of both children with enthusiasm.

As the years passed, Virginia accepted extra shifts eagerly. In order to provide for her family, she often worked more than sixty hours per week. She reasoned that overtime pay was so much higher than what Lee could earn, he was better off running the household.

Shortly after Bobby had started kindergarten and Bart the third grade, Virginia arrived home anticipating her usual mammoth breakfast, only to discover her husband absent. Hours later he appeared, slightly drunk, having been out partying all night. He denied wrongdoing, insisted he had earned the diversion and voiced resentment at her questions and accusations.

The spiral had begun. Lee's absences grew more frequent and male visitors often dropped by their apartment. Virginia found an overnight babysitter necessary for her own peace of mind. The expenses increased, the frustrations increased and her weight increased. Lee compensated for his failings by providing appetizing meals. His wife carried a feast that was the envy of her co-workers to work every night and consumed every morsel. She continued to devour multi-liter bottles of Pepsi with every shift, ostensibly to stay awake. She never mentioned the problems at home, always presenting a picture of domestic bliss.

Despite the deterioration of her personal life, Virginia delivered exemplary work as a paramedic and received commendations and promotions as a result. As her weight increased, the company transferred her to dispatch. She also taught classes in Advanced Cardiac Life Support to the other EMTs, making herself a valued member of the team. Always affable, her cheery laugh and easy manner reassured her co-workers and subordinates. Her willingness to work long hours without complaint endeared her to her superiors who were all too willing to overlook her burgeoning bulk. In a later attempt at explaining these voluntary long hours, Virginia admitted that she felt in control and comfortable only when in her work situation.

Bart grew to manhood as a responsible and serious individual. His grades and behavior at school were excellent. When he graduated from high school, he enlisted in the Marines and continued to be the great pride of his mother's life. Her other son, Bobby, challenged the system and his mother's efforts at discipline with every turn, always certain of his father's backing. Virginia dealt with his minor scrapes with the law, frequent bouts of underage drinking and drug abuse. Bobby's stay at a rehabilitation hospital left her in debt. Bart attempted to be supportive of his mother from afar while Bobby undermined what scant self-esteem she held. Lee continued in his lifestyle, apparently oblivious to his wife's distress.

Home on leave, Bart was aghast to see the decline in his mother. Confronting her with his serious concern about her deteriorating health, Bart convinced Virginia to investigate gastric surgery. More to placate her persistent child than through a concern over her own welfare, she met with a bariatric physician.

Weighing 430 pounds at just over five feet in height and confined to a wheelchair for mobility, Virginia remembers being unable to scale even the curb to the sidewalk at the hospital. Because of the nature of her position, she was able to perform her duties from the chair. With a blasé attitude presented to her friends, she harbored dread of losing her sole coping mechanism, food. Her husband finally voiced support and promised to tailor his culinary offerings to suit her anticipated needs after surgery.

Of the team appointed to prepare Virginia for surgery, only the psychologist expressed reservations. He required a commitment from the prospective patient of weekly therapy sessions for a minimum of one year after surgery. Accurately assessing her personal struggles as the cause of her excessive intake, he feared replacement behaviors would occur if she didn't ferret out the source of her unhappiness and deal successfully with it. Virginia agreed, recognizing that psychological changes were imperative for her physical well-being.

A Roux n Y procedure was performed and the post-operative course was uneventful. Virginia's hospital room overflowed with plants and flowers, cards and visitors. Her eldest son, home again on leave, provided support by his presence and Lee stood his vigil at the bedside. Bobby was absent.

In the months that followed, Virginia's weight dropped markedly. With the aid of the bariatric support group and the psychologist, her self-image soared. She worked diligently to bargain with her demons. Constant reinforcement from her son, physicians and co-workers provided support for the task.

When interviewed, Virginia had trimmed 200 pounds from her frame. Although still markedly heavy, she happily reported being able to step up on the curb at the hospital. The wheelchair had been discarded and, for the first time in her life, she joined a bowling league. Her infectious laugh hinted at inner contentment. She continued to meet the appointments with the psychologist and managed to establish some behavioral contracts with her husband. She would no longer tolerate coming home to his stranger visitors and he agreed to her stipulations. Bart pressed her to end the marriage and move on but she claimed a sense of responsibility toward her husband and refused to consider the possibility.

Virginia's goals are travel, shedding another hundred pounds and continuing therapy. The constant smiles and sunny disposition she presents to the world are no longer facades. She is looking forward to Bart's approaching wedding and shopping for just the right dress for the occasion. Because of gastric surgery and adjunct therapies, her future appears brighter than her past.

Chapter 8
Lynda

The term "caregiver" defined Lynda's personality. The oldest of four and the only girl, she shouldered the burdens of childcare, meal preparation and maintenance of a household when herself a child. Her mother worked as a nurse in the evenings and her father held down two jobs. Her sense of responsibility for her surroundings and those around her overwhelmed her and resulted in an existence fraught with frustration, acquiescence and morbid obesity.

Partially as an escape from the confines of her home, Lynda entered nurses' training and began to nurture strangers. Immediately after completion of her studies, she and a number of fellow graduates accepted travel assignments, ostensibly to 'see the world' but in Lynda's case to forsake the obligations assigned to her by her family. Unrecognized, the psychological baggage endowed by her parents followed her and was to plague her for the remainder of her life.

Working in the Emergency Department of a small hospital in rural Louisiana, Lynda met and married a dashing young police officer who frequently dropped by for coffee or a chat in the middle of her night shift. The fact that he bore responsibility for the upbringing of his four young boys didn't deter her in the least and she cheerfully embraced them as her own. Marrying into an Italian-American family and desperate for its approval, Lynda's escalation of food intake began. Sundays were celebrated with massive dinners served after church to the extended gathering. Spaghetti with lots of cheeses, fried chicken hot from the skillet, hams and succulent local specialties topped the list of offerings accompanied by myriad vegetables, breads, salads and wonderful desserts. Lynda ate along with the family when she wasn't hungry because she thought this would gain her approval. Before long, she and her hearty husband were carrying the evidence of their indulgences.

Her first pregnancy and the severe illness of her new father-in-law coupled to trigger a culinary compulsion for Lynda and she rose to the occasion. Her metabolism naturally slowed during the development of the child but her appetite and need for self-nurturing did not. During that same time, she would visit her ailing in-law and share hot French bread with loads of butter and jam as a ritual. The arrival of her daughter into the brood of boys was heralded by all. Delighted with her baby, the young mother slept less, ate more, and continued to work full-time. Additionally, she parented a boisterous household and, true to her regimented upbringing, kept an immaculate house.

Her husband loved to cook and Lynda gladly relinquished the daily task to him. As his family grew, the food bill climbed and his expertise in the kitchen sharpened. The boys arrived home from school anticipating a robust meal and were never disappointed. Dinner became a time of happiness and sharing. Both Lynda and her husband partook freely of the bounty prepared and carried increasingly more weight on their frames.

A second child of her own followed for Lynda and the weight gaining experience was repeated. Having never lost the additional pounds from her earlier pregnancy, she left the hospital at 260 pounds with yet another baby boy. Happy, from her own description, she and her husband relished the demands of their growing family and celebrated each blissful moment with food.

Through the children's developmental years, Lynda continued to carry the burden of home-maker, mother and nurse. She accepted and devoted her energies to each. At the hospital, she agreed to act as the manager of critical care, encompassing a busy Emergency Department and active Intensive Care Unit. Unable to face conflict or tolerate perceived antagonism from anyone, she balanced the needs of her staff with the dictates of administration, often at her own emotional expense. As a result of her need to mediate instead of command, insignificant differences in opinion escalated between her employees. Strong, aggressive staff nurses achieved their self-serving goals and others, disgruntled, left for alternative employment.

With the children essentially grown, Lynda should have enjoyed the time that she and her husband had worked toward. Rather, physical problems began to plague both of them. He was diagnosed with adult onset diabetes, the price paid for a lifetime of unchecked intake and morbid obesity. She noted uncomfortable swelling in her legs on a daily basis. Walking the length of the hall at the hospital required effort, triggered knee pain and left her short of breath. Despondent over the deterioration of her body, Lynda cried into the five pillows she needed for comfort during her sleeping hours.

When her husband announced he was contemplating the frequently advertised gastric surgery to interrupt his uncontrollable need to eat, Lynda was surprised. He had never mentioned the possibility. Frightened for his health as well as her own, she quickly agreed to meet with the surgeon to confer about the operative possibility. After discussing surgery, viewing descriptive tapes, attending group meetings and getting insurance approval, her husband had the procedure. Originally, the two had requested surgery at the same time but the surgeon had dissuaded Lynda from this course of action, citing her husband's medical problems as the most pressing. Accepting that she might also be needed to care for him after surgery, she again acquiesced.

The surgery was a huge success and Lynda's husband adapted well to the constraints on his intake. Three weeks after surgery, he no longer needed daily injections of insulin and was able to discard all medication within three months. Encouraged by his steady weight loss and enthusiastic support, Lynda wholeheartedly followed his footsteps.

Although her insurance carrier had approved the surgery, Lynda's employer was less than enthusiastic. A leave was granted after she, uncharacteristically, threatened to resign if the time off wasn't granted. Two weeks after the surgery, she began to get calls from her staff at home. They were overworked from an unusually heavy load at the hospital. Numerous complaints and gripes were reported to her several times a day and she brooded over them long after the phone calls. In an effort to stem the discontent, she returned to work early. Hoping that her presence would be perceived as supportive and self-sacrificial, she was dismayed to find the problems seemed to mushroom when she was available to listen.

During this time period, the eldest son married and moved his new wife in with the family. A diagnosed paranoid schizophrenic, the child had always required a great deal of monitoring to insure adherence to his medication regimen. Thrilled that he had married and seemed to have a life of normalcy ahead, the parents welcomed his new bride into their home. Within weeks, Lynda was silently fretting over the situation. Not only was the additional member of family unwilling to help with the household chores, she actually increased Lynda's work load. Always an immaculate housekeeper, she cleaned after the family and dropped into bed long after everyone else was asleep. Piles of dirty clothes were regularly placed near the washing machine and Lynda begrudgingly washed, folded and put away each piece.

With demands being made on her time from every front, Lynda neglected the frequent small meals she was required to consume to maintain her health. Entire days at the hospital would pass without a morsel of food or a taste of soup. Evenings brought precious little time to take in the tiny bites she needed. Her husband recognized that she wasn't eating and prepared foods especially for her and tried to monitor her intake.

She erroneously reported successful progress to her doctors at her regular visits. The weight loss was steady and she attributed the fatigue to the demands of her job. She quit going to the bariatric support group meetings, justifying her absences by other claims on her time.

Eight months after surgery, she was experiencing weariness that pressed to her bones. Leaving the house before her husband and falling into bed before he arrived home, she didn't acknowledge the magnitude of her anorexia. Clumps of hair on her pillow were disregarded and she gamely continued to juggle the challenges of nursing management and an unruly household. The weight loss persisted and Lynda shoved big uniforms to the back of her closet, pledging to organize and donate as soon as she had the energy.

Only after a staff member threatened to call Lynda's physician did she submit to blood chemistry tests to assess the actual status of her health. Every single value was labeled either "high" or "low" as compared to normal levels. She appeared defeated, worn and depleted. When she wanted to cross one leg over the other, she had to lift the leg with her hands. Her abdomen was swollen from a liver enlarged from starvation. Her legs and feet were grossly swollen with edema. Against her wishes, she was hospitalized immediately.

Because of the negligible intake, the pouch portion of her stomach had shrunk and would require frequent intake challenges to attain its former capacity. Dieticians at the hospital prepared palatable, digestible nourishment for Lynda and a nurse was assigned to monitor her intake during each of six meals a day. At first, she vomited everything she attempted to eat and refused to try. With the encouragement of the surgeon and a stern directive from her husband, she began to take and retain small amounts of food. Protein powder was sprinkled on everything and icy Ensure was instantly available for sipping. Follow-up blood work revealed no improvement.

In order to save her life, the surgeon inserted a central intravenous line so that nutrition could be provided while Lynda learned to eat again. Each evening, she attached herself to an additive-rich concoction and discontinued the infusion in the morning. Slowly, the liver failure reversed, the edema lessened and the fatigue abated. After three months of the intravenous therapy and steadily increasing oral intake, the central line was removed.

With regular professional psychological support, Lynda was able to identify and alter the contributing factors of her near death experience. With her husband's encouragement, she informed her son and daughter-in-law that they were responsible for their own household chores, including cooking and cleaning. A deadline was set for them to establish their own residence. She structured regular interval breaks at work for small snacks. She occasionally unplugged the telephone at home if the work-related calls became incessant and frustrating. After a lifetime of placing her needs behind those of all others, Lynda was learning to move herself up in the line. The loss of 160 pounds and the pleasure of slipping into a size 10 dress were causes for celebration but the real victory came when Lynda realized she had discovered herself.

Chapter 9

The Doctor

Before a personal decision committing to surgery has been reached, a consultation with a prospective surgeon needs to be arranged. Integral to the success of the procedure, the choice of the surgeon demands careful consideration. The operation of choice, VBG or gastric bypass, must be performed by a skilled practitioner who has experience in the techniques required and has been trained in the specifics of bariatric procedures. To insure the greatest possibility for patient success, the surgeon's efforts should be supported by a medical bariatric specialist who will provide long-term surveillance, including monitoring of nutritional status and the progress or remission of any pre-operative medical conditions.

Billboards and newspaper advertisements tout the marvelous weight loss results achieved with surgery performed by a specific physician or group of physicians. Although this is good in that it attracts attention, better methods of locating a bariatric surgeon are available. Assuredly, many competent doctors advertise but other referral sources are often more effective in locating a practitioner with the expertise desired. A referral from a physician, nurse or other medical professional who has witnessed the progress of bariatric patients under the care of a particular surgeon can provide an accurate testimonial. The value of a positive referral from a patient who has undergone either the VBG or a gastric bypass reinforces either advertisement or medical endorsement. A recommendation by someone who has passed through the experience can do much to allay the prospective candidate's fears.

Because of the importance of follow-up by the surgeon, one should be chosen with a practice geographically located near the patient to provide access for periodic evaluation appointments and emergency care if needed. If the surgeon of choice practices in an area remote to the patient, another practitioner must be established as local, back-up support. This step should be accomplished before any procedure is undertaken and with the approval of the operative physician.

In the USA, confirmation of the credentials of a prospective surgeon or a referral can be obtained by contacting:

The American Society for Bariatric Surgery
140 N.W. 75th Drive
Suite C
Gainesville, FL 32607

When first interviewing the physician and discussing the possibility of surgery, the patient needs to voice his many concerns. The perceptive physician welcomes the opportunity to clarify any misconceptions and provide information. Among the questions to consider are the following:

1. Which surgery is right for me?

    Complete with illustrations, the physician will describe the changes proposed for your gastro-intestinal tract to achieve the goals of limited intake and significant weight loss. Specific to your needs, he will explain the rationale for the choice of procedure.

2. Who will assist the surgeon during the procedure?

    Many physicians employ surgical nurses or operating technicians to assist in surgery and these individuals often function much as a second physician would, so familiar are they with the equipment and techniques used by the surgeon. In some cases, another surgeon will be asked to assist.

3. How many procedures has the surgeon performed?

   Knowing the number of times the practitioner has performed the operation gives the patient an indication not only of familiarity with the procedure but is also a reflection of his commitment to helping the morbidly obese through surgical means.

4. What is the complication rate among the surgeon's previous bariatric patients?

   The ethical surgeon will disclose this information. To gain further details of consequence, the nature of complications should be queried. With a range from nausea and/or vomiting, not an unusual occurrence, to life-threatening peritonitis, the character of the complications provides more information than the actual number.

5. Where will be the surgery be performed?

   The proper equipment and personnel to provide peri-operative care is a mandatory qualification for a facility, usually a hospital, to be chosen for the procedure. Just as the surgeon is expected to be experienced in the surgery, the hospital team should be skilled in the care of the bariatric patient. Accommodation for patients who incur critical complications is essential. Pharmacy, respiratory therapy and nursing all fulfill vital roles in attaining the successful surgical outcome.

6. Ask for a description of the peri-operative support team.

   As has been previously discussed, members of the support team include a nutritional specialist, physical therapist, psychological counselor and medical management physician. The purpose of the support team is to increase the patient's chance of a successful outcome. Recognizing the importance of the group, the surgeon will have the adjunctive staff identified and in place well before the operation.

7. Request a meeting with one or more of the surgeon's previous bariatric patients.

   The surgeon, after speaking with the potential candidate for a procedure, will provide the name of a patient who would be willing to share his or her surgical experience with you.

   Where possible, the person would have had the same surgery contemplated by the inquiring individual and will be able to provide insights not available from any other source. If the prospective surgeon is unable or unwilling to suggest a patient for your interview, consider that hesitation a "red flag" danger signal and delve further into the physician's record of success or seek an alternate physician.

8. How will I pay for the procedure?

   In the face of mounting costs due to serious health problems in the morbidly obese, insurance carriers often consider bariatric surgery in a positive light. Strong advocacy and complete documentation from a primary physician will be helpful in obtaining approval for a procedure.

   If you don't have insurance, other avenues are open to you. Contact a university teaching hospital near you and discover if bariatric procedures are being performed. All the questions listed above carry increased importance in the teaching environment. Do not consider allowing a procedure to be performed if the surgeon has no experience and minimal training. If at all possible, schedule the operation for one of the months of April, May or June, and request the surgery be done by a staff surgeon and the chief surgical resident. With the years of his training coming to a close, the chief resident offers the highest degree of expertise and knowledge of any of the student doctors. The staff surgeon provides guidance and support to the residents during the actual procedure and during the hospitalization.

One of the greatest difficulties in this environment is the absence of a consistent team for follow-up. Due to the rotational nature of teaching hospital staffs, the possibility exists of never seeing the same physician twice. To overcome that handicap, it becomes especially important that the patient is well-informed. It is always appropriate for the patient to ask questions and any concerns that arise must be addressed immediately. Before committing to bariatric surgery at a teaching hospital, request that a permanent contact person be appointed. A nurse, dietician or other sympathetic individual can help you navigate the sometimes perplexing medical maze leading to your goal.

Help is available from supportive organizations. The websites at the end of this book are only a few of the many that provide encouragement, information and support.

Chapter 10

The Event

The series of events surrounding surgery can be daunting. Unforeseen examinations, sensations and expenses can cause unnecessary fear and intimidation for the patient confronting a bariatric procedure. Preparation and education erase many of those anxieties and serve to make the encounter as pleasant as possible. To complement the information provided by the patient's personal physician, the following description offers insight into a typical operative experience.

Referral to a surgeon by the prospective patient's primary physician initiates the process and marks the beginning of a satisfying relationship.

My name is Susan. I am fifty years old and have been heavy my entire life. I felt good up until the last year before my surgery. Then I started to have headaches and I had no energy. I went to see my doctor and he found high blood pressure and an enlarged heart. He suggested I think about having surgery so I wouldn't eat so much. After talking with my family, I made an appointment with the surgeon he recommended. Truthfully, I would never have even thought of having the surgery if my health wasn't affected. I was so afraid to die and miss out on my grandchildren growing up.

I weighed 324 pounds when I went to see Dr. Brown. My medical doctor had sent copies of all my records and the results of the tests ahead so she would be familiar with my case. She visited with me for a long time and explained the operation. She told me she did three or four surgeries a week and showed me pictures of some of her patients after they lost weight. I wasn't nearly as nervous after I left her office.

One of her office workers talked to me about the cost of the surgery. Luckily, my insurance approved the operation and I could afford it.

Mandatory attendance at one or more group meetings of actual and potential bariatric patients must be completed before the procedure. In this manner, the prospective patient enjoys the opportunity of talking with others having endured the trials of morbid obesity and chosen the ultimate treatment modern medicine offers. Establishing a support system external from family and friends provides a sense of emotional stability and a greater likelihood of successful adjustment after surgery.

Somehow, I expected the members of the group to be critical of me. I was so miserable. My clothes were handmade tents and I didn't wear make-up because I just didn't feel like trying to look good. I dreaded going in there and being with the slim people who had gone through the surgery.

There were maybe twenty people there that first night. I felt right at home from the start. Sure, some were normal sized but several were bigger than me. They knew what I was going through like no one else. They had been in the supermarket and had kids point and laugh and look in the basket. Each one told the same story in a different way. We related.

Dr. Brown came and spent time with any of us who wanted her to. The speaker was a dietician who talked about...well, food. As I remember, she told us about the importance of fiber in our diets both before the surgery and afterward. She pointed out that foods high in fiber took longer to digest and it took longer to get hungry. She gave us a list of those foods we needed to consider and ways of preparing them that were easy and nutritious. The dietician spoke at every meeting and talked about a different food group each time. She encouraged all of us to call her with questions.

Dr. Brown told me I needed to go to four meetings before she would do surgery. The group met once a month at her hospital. I didn't mind going at all and looked forward to seeing my new friends.

A psychological evaluation must be done prior to the surgery to ascertain the level of patient commitment and the psychological readiness of the patient. The psychiatrist, psychologist or social worker chosen will also offer a choice of alternative coping mechanisms designed to facilitate the transition from an obese person to a much thinner one, the change from using food as a crutch to viewing the bounty as nourishment only.

> Surprise! Surprise! The social worker was a big gal, too. She wasn't as large as I was when I went for my evaluation but big enough that she made me feel better. She and I talked for a couple of hours about how much I ate, when I ate and why I ate.

Ascertaining the amount of food taken on a daily basis provides indications of behavioral vs metabolic components to the patient's addiction. An estimate of projected weight loss after surgery reaches a higher level of accuracy when this information is provided. Additionally, the patient often denies the magnitude of the addiction before measuring the quantities of intake prior to the surgery. The mental health care provider may suggest journaling to achieve the precision desired.

Identifying the time of day of greatest intake allows the counselor to assist in tailoring new coping mechanisms for individual patients. Cognizant of time triggers that signal potential problem zones, the patient knowledgeably approaches those hours armed with positive anticipation and firm plans to avert personal frustration.

Determination of the motivation behind food addiction often requires a series of sessions with the professional and entails true resolve from the prospective patient. The answers might be transparent and easily identified or hidden from insight, demanding considerable effort to expose. In either case, revelation of the causes of food addiction smoothes the way for emotional as well as physical success in weight loss following surgery.

> We talked about my relationship with my husband and kids and what they thought about the surgery. Mainly, we talked about the change in my life that was coming and how I felt about that. I told her that I was really scared and wasn't sure I was doing the right thing but I wanted to live a long life.
>
> She spoke with such a soft voice, I had trouble hearing her some of the time. Of course, I did most of the talking, anyway! [Susan laughs heartily]. She told me to call her any time I had questions or problems and even gave me the number to her beeper! After she told me she had given the go-ahead for my operation, I was thrilled.

In the days immediately prior to the procedure, pre-operative laboratory work will be done as well as a chest x-ray and electrocardiogram. The pathology of severe obesity predisposes to liver disease, respiratory ailments, high blood pressure, heart disease and skeletal injury due to the extreme taxation on the body caused by the excess weight. In order to accurately evaluate the extent of damage done to the body's systems and correct the consequences whenever possible to assure the greatest possibility for a complication-free procedure, current data is necessary.

> No one likes getting stuck with a needle but I could hardly wait. I knew that the blood tests were the last thing to be done before my big day. I wore that bandaid proudly that night!

The stomach must be entirely empty for the procedure. Anesthesia cannot be administered if retained gastric contents are suspected because of the possibility of aspiration into the lungs. Life-threatening pneumonia can result and prolong hospitalization. In addition, minimizing gastric contents provides the surgeon with an ideal area for his work.

> Just to be on the safe side, I quit eating or drinking after supper the night before the surgery. Dr. Brown said I could drink water until midnight but none after. I was awake most of the night, partly from nervousness and partly from excitement, but I never drank a drop.

Admission to the hospital on the day of surgery should be done promptly to allow the anesthesiologist and the surgery crew enough time for preparation. Often, personal information including social security number, date of birth, emergency contact person and phone numbers as well as an arrangement of payment choice will have been completed in advance, minimizing the time needed in the actual admissions office. If consents for treatment have been previously completed in the physician's office, copies and the original will be included in the file and further decrease the duration of time needed for paperwork.

My husband and I arrived at six in the morning, almost an hour before we were supposed to. The clerk was so cheerful and wished me luck after we signed in. A nurse came and got us and took us into a little room to get me ready. I had to take off all of my clothes and put on one of those skimpy gowns. I was given a fluffy blue hat to cover my hair. After that, everything went pretty fast.

The anesthesiologist came in and asked the same questions as my other doctors. He had some trouble finding a vein but finally got an IV in my arm and told me he would make sure I was comfortable. The nurse gave me a drug through the IV and I don't remember a thing after that. My husband tells me he was asked to wait in the visitor's lounge from then on.

The length of the procedure depends upon the specific operation performed, the speed of the surgeon and the number of complications encountered (if any). The sleeping patient will be meticulously monitored by the anesthesia staff for detection of any respiratory difficulties, adverse reaction to the anesthetic agents or episodic abnormal pulse or blood pressure. Poor visualization of the operative site due to an unusually excessive layer of fat will increase the operative time as will any bleeding abnormalities or unforeseen technical problems. Prior to the procedure, the surgeon will advise those who will be waiting of an approximate time frame and the surgical staff will provide periodic reports of the patient's progress.

Upon successful completion of the procedure, the patient will be transported from the surgical suite to the post-anesthesia care unit, commonly called the recovery room. Careful monitoring of vital signs and levels of consciousness will be watched and treated as needed by trained personnel. Discharge from the recovery room to a patient room follows full responsiveness. Intravenous infusions will be continued because of the necessity for the patient to take nothing by mouth. A urinary catheter, inserted during surgery, remains for a short period of time after the operation until the patient is able to walk to the bathroom.

Waking up after surgery is like clearing cobwebs from your brain. A few are whisked away at a time until you can see and hear and talk. The pain wasn't bad at first but as I woke up, the burning in my belly got worse. The nurse gave me a shot of Demerol and that helped a lot. As soon as I felt like it, my husband was allowed in to see me. He was so relieved, he kept squeezing my hand and kissing my forehead.

My mouth was dry from the anesthesia. I was given a little sponge stick soaked in ice water to suck on and that was heaven! After I moved to my room, I slept most of the day.

The first time I got out of bed, I thought my stomach would burst! I was so weak that two nurses and my husband had to help while I held a pillow to my incision. The pillow seemed to help the pain. Each time was easier and by the second day, I could get up by myself. The nurses gave me pain injections when I asked for them but I didn't take a lot.

The nurses would insist I cough every so often and I used the pillow on my incision for that, too. Dr. Brown had ordered respiratory treatments several times a day to make sure I didn't have any problems with my lungs.

The length of hospitalization depends upon the type of surgery, the patient's response and the physician's wishes.

> I did so well that Dr. Brown discharged me in three days. I couldn't wait to see my babies. She sent me home with prescriptions for antibiotics and liquid pain medicine but I never needed it.

The first oral intake is provided approximately 24 hours after the procedure. Clear liquids will be offered first and thicker liquids next. The dietician and surgeon will advise how quickly to advance the intake. The anticipated progression of liquid to foods will have been discussed prior to surgery and written copies of recommended nutrition furnished. Ready availability of appropriate foods in the hospital is to be expected but having an array of palatable and well-tolerated grocery products in the home setting entails planning.

> The first thing I put in my mouth was diet red gelatin, the kind with no sugar. I felt it on my tongue, cool and slippery, before it melted and I swallowed. I can't ever remember tasting, really tasting, gelatin before. I expected some nausea and there was just a passing queasiness. I didn't want any more, just that one taste.
>
> Before the doctor would stop the IV, I had to prove I would drink enough. So, I sipped and sipped on water. I really prefer soft drinks but those

were forbidden because of the carbonation. She said I was doing well enough on the second day that the IV was removed. The most difficult part was taking the vitamins. The liquid went down easily enough but the taste was bad. I was allowed to suck on sugar-free mints afterward to kill the taste.

Before leaving the hospital, the patient and a caregiver will be taught wound care. The incision should be cleaned and painted with an antiseptic once a day until the physician is satisfied all potential for local infection is gone.

My incision was closed with great, big wires covered with rubber tubes. My husband really didn't want to help take care of it but the nurse insisted he learn how to clean the area. After we went home, he helped me every evening after my shower and told me every single time that my stomach was getting smaller. I think, secretly, he was proud to be a part of my getting better. Dr. Brown took out half of the stitches in two weeks and the other half the week after that. We watched it and never saw any redness or drainage.

Weight loss is rapid in the first few weeks and months after surgery. Although sweets are poorly tolerated, other high calorie foods will prevent the patient from shedding the maximum number of pounds. Monitoring of the types and amounts of food will be overseen by a dietician but ultimately, the patient is responsible.

I lost 12 pounds the first week. What a wonderful feeling. The weight didn't come off as fast after I started eating soft foods and I had to be real careful. Mashed potatoes and gravy, cream of chicken soup and guacamole are the favorites that I had to eat in very small portions. After a few months, I could eat almost anything I wanted if I chewed well before swallowing and took small bites.

My surgery was 19 months ago and I now weigh 182 pounds. My blood pressure is normal and the doctor says my heart is fine. I walk every day and love waking up in the morning. My family and friends are my cheerleaders and my grandkids give me high fives and tell me how good I look.

Dr. Brown discharged me from her care after four months and now I see my medical doctor for tests on my blood every six months. I still go to group meetings and visit the hospital when someone else is having the surgery.

Would I do it again? In a heartbeat.

Chapter 11
Aftermath

In the months and years following surgery for severe obesity, expected and unexpected changes occur to those having made the decision. Psychological adjustment is necessary to cope with the physical differences, even though they are desirable and anticipated: an alien image is being presented to the self and others. As tightly bound as the proverbial "white on rice", body and attitudinal adaptations must be made for optimal success. In the following examples, offered by actual bariatric patients, the intertwining of the two and the fragile balance achieved become evident.

Harold responds to the query regarding the changes he has experienced in the three years since surgery and a weight loss of 260 pounds. Hal, aged 50, lives in the western part of the United States and works for the government. A gregarious and warm individual, Hal previously was employed in sales and various aspects of radio broadcasting. Widowed and childless, he has rediscovered an active social life.

I would have to say that prior to surgery, I thought I didn't live life as a fat person. I went out, kept a job and had several careers, dated, got married, had friends and just lived what I thought was a normal life. I wasn't a guy in a house that had to be destroyed to get me out and to a hospital. I now realize that psychologically, I had also accepted a fat person's mentality. I made excuses and adjustments in my thinking about things I had difficulty doing or wanted to do. I was able to navigate between the two mindsets. In my mind's eye, I never saw the fat.

Only when my health began to fail did I consider such a drastic remedy.

After the surgery and recovery period, I was amazed at the changes I saw, both in myself and others. Immediately, I was perceived to be more assertive, not as "nice" as people thought I was before. Others stood closer to me and paid more attention to my opinions.

I had always prided myself on dressing well but when I dropped from a size 68 to a size 36, I became a clothes horse. One of the really weird things was that I became physically attractive and I truly didn't know how to react to flirtation by females – it had never happened to me before.

I was extremely weak after the surgery and had some complications and vowed never to feel that way again. I joined a gym, began working out and discovered that I enjoyed it.

There were many small discoveries every day that were unnerving. I had to mourn the loss of my best friend, food. I could no longer abuse it and that frustrated me, many times to tears.

The physical recuperation following surgery was grueling for me. No one, except for other bypass patients, can understand how many physical, mental and emotional changes bombard you after the surgery.

There were also small, personal victory moments. I was thrilled when I could buckle a regular airline seatbelt around myself. To be able to clean myself after using the toilet without resorting to a shower was a bonus. A bigger victory was being able to throw away the insulin syringes. My shirtfronts were no longer spotted with dropped food. I no longer needed to rent full-sized cars or have a king-sized bed.

I knew I no longer looked fat when children stopped staring at me in stores or on the street.

I see someone the size I used to be and it makes me sad. I want to reach out and tell him that he doesn't have to suffer but I refrain, it's none of my business.

Some incidents are fun. Having someone you've known for years walk right by you because you look so different is mind-blowing.

It takes a long time to stop being fat in your mind. I remember the moment I stopped being a fat person very clearly. I was taking a hand-to-hand combat class at the police academy and was chosen to perform a stunt where I would take a blow, then fall to the ground. As I prepared to take the fall, I was afraid I wouldn't be able to get up, embarrassing myself. After the fall, I got up quickly and in that moment, realized I was no longer obese.

Alana tells a different tale but an implication of the significance of the physical/psychological coupling resounds. Preferring to remain anonymous regarding her personal information, she offers insight into her post-operative experience.

Things haven't gone so well for me. I'm almost two years post operative and have only lost 80 pounds. Not very impressive. The psychological aspects following the surgery have been horrible. I keep second guessing myself, wondering if I was responsible for screwing up a surgical weight loss procedure. I beat myself up all the time.

I'm going to try again. Hopefully things will turn out better the second time around. The majority of people do terrific. Why couldn't I?

Barbara, who also prefers no personal information be given, describes her experience.

Like many obese people, I grew up an overweight child. I was the constant subject of teasing and torment through high school. I managed to stay around 190 pounds since the fifth grade. I went to college and was very active in school activities. However, I just couldn't manage to lose any weight. I tried every program, every product, every deterrent on the market. I would lose a few pounds then gain it back and more.

I met a wonderful man and we were married two years later. Then I started gaining more weight. I ballooned up to 276 pounds. I have back problems and it was impossible to walk, stand or even sit comfortably. I begged my doctors to help me and give me some of the new prescription drugs but none would. I am 26 years old.

Then, my sister, who is also obese, shared that she was investigating gastric bypass surgery. I was initially very wary of this but agreed to go to informational meetings at the hospital. Those meetings changed my outlook. After insurance approval, we both had our surgeries on the same day.

Immediately after surgery, I was a bit down. I would cry at the drop of a hat. I had lost my best friend, food. I could no longer turn to this "friend" for comfort when things went wrong. I couldn't eat a bag of chips, a carton of milk or a huge bowl of chocolate ice cream. I had to confront the issues in my life. From doing that, I saved my failing marriage.

I can easily say that this surgery saved my life. I am so much happier now. I look forward to doing things. I enjoy walking or biking. I am no longer too tired to do anything but sit in front of the television. I smile more, people hold doors open for me and I notice they don't stare anymore. It's a wonderful thing to feel "normal". I have lost 105 pounds and have only 25 pounds more to reach my goal. My sister has lost 130 pounds.

I don't miss chocolate, breads or sweet things. I am completely satisfied after a small meal (typically between a half to a third of a cup of food). I try to have a protein drink for breakfast and have to give myself a B12 shot every month but it's a good tradeoff.

I have never regretted my decision at all.

Charles adds his narrative. A Vietnam war veteran, Chuck retired from governmental service and is currently self-employed. Married with three adult children and one grandchild, he boasts a 207 pound weight loss over sixteen months. His interests include boating and remaining active in service organizations.

I personally think the psychological adjustments had to take place prior to the operation. I spent quite a bit of time contacting others who have had the procedure and spent hours talking with them to find out what to expect and how they felt about the process following the operation. I knew in advance what to look forward to and not too much came as a surprise.

One major point was that not one of the seven I contacted regretted having it done and all of them would have it done again. This included one who had major surgical and post-surgical difficulties.

The fact that I wouldn't be able to tolerate some foods did not come as a surprise. I was ready for the adjustment. Most of those I contacted warned me that I would not be able to eat some foods and I appreciated their honesty.

One of the hardest adjustments was learning to eat in public and at family gatherings. I always loved the holidays and all the good food. As a result, it was difficult to pass on most of them and just limit myself to a small taste but I did and it worked out fine.

Another thing that takes a while to get used to is self-permission to leave food on my plate. I found that I could ask the waitperson to omit the items that I knew I could not eat. Often, when my wife and I would go out to eat, she would order a little more than she wanted and we would split the entrée. When I explained to the waitperson the reason, they had no problem and would often place a small portion on a separate plate before bringing it to the table.

Shrinking is a problem, albeit a good one, which must be faced. At first I would have my clothes altered. But, then, two months later, they were too big again. After a while, I only had a couple of pieces altered and then finally, began to buy new clothes. That was a tremendous psychological booster.

I really think having the operation was harder on my wife than it was on me. She had to learn to cook all over again and she would try to avoid those things she knew I couldn't handle. As often as I told her it didn't bother me for her to eat steak while I enjoyed my soup, I know it bothered her. She loves hamburgers so every once in a while, I just go out and get her a burger and bring it home for her. Otherwise, she wouldn't ever eat them.

When eating out socially, it is a trick to only eat a bite or two of salad and skip the bread plate but it can be done and works well. One must enjoy the company and conversation and focus on those instead of the food.

I suppose that when all is said and done, the biggest psychological adjustment is to realize that for the first time in your life, you eat to live instead of live to eat. It works and I feel good.

Tremendous psychological adjustments must be made to accept a new self. Knowledge and flexibility are key to acceptance and ultimate success. As evidenced by those who shared their stories, gastric surgery can and does change lives. Finally, as Chuck Woodward adds:

Be good to yourself. You are truly your own best friend.

Endnotes

1. The Third National Health and Nutrition Examination Survey (1988-1994), National Center for Health Statistics of the Center for Disease Control of the United States. Website: www.cdc.gov/NCHS/products/catalogs/subject/NHANES3/NHANES3.HTM.

2. The Third National Health and Nutrition Examination Survey.

3. The Third National Health and Nutrition Examination Survey.

4. American Society for Bariatric Surgery website 1999.

5. Choban *et al.* 1999, page 491.

6. Choban *et al.* 1999, page 491

7. Choban *et al.* 1999, page 494.

8. Choban *et al.* 1999, page 494.

9. Choban *et al.* 1999, page 494.

10. Choban *et al.* 1999, page 494.

11. Bessler 1999 conference summary.

12. Bessler 1999 conference summary.

13. Choban *et al.* 1999, page 494.

14. Choban *et al.* 1999, page 494.

15. Bessler 1999, conference summary.

16. www.obesitylapbandsurgery.com. 1998, page 2.

17. www.obesitylapbandsurgery.com. 1998, page 2.

18. Wright 1998, page 2.

19. www.Asbs.org/html/story_4.html, page 2.

20. www.nwobese.com/gastric.html, page 1.

21. www.drchampion.com/rny.htm.

22. www.Asbs.org/html/ration.html.

23. www.Asbs.org/html/ration.html.

24. Bessler 1999, page 5.

25. www.Asbs.org/html/ration.html.

26. www.Asbs.org/html/ration.html.

Bibliography

American Society for Bariatric Surgery Website 'Rationale for the Surgical Treatment of Morbid Obesity' p. 10 www.asbs.org

Bessler, Mark, M.D. 1999. 'Multidisciplinary Management of Obesity', 85th Clinical Congress of the American College of Surgeons.

Brolin, Robert, Bradley, Lisa J. and Taliwal, Rajiv V. (1998) 'Unsuspected Cirrhosis Discovered During Elective Obesity Operations', *Archives of Surgery*, *133* 84–88.

Choban, Patricia, & Anyejekwe, Jacqueline, Burge, Jean C. and Flanebaum, Louis, (1999) 'Health Status Assessment of the Impact of Weight Loss Following Roux-en-Y Gastric Bypass for Clinically Severe Obesity', *Journal of the American College of Surgeons, 188* 5, 491–496.

Cowley, Geoffrey and Begley, Sharon, (2000) 'Fat For Life?', *Newsweek*, July 3, pp. 40–47.

Curry, Thomas, and Carter, Preston, Porter, Clifford A., Watts, David M. (1998) 'Resectional Gastric Bypass Is a New Alternative in Morbid Obesity', *The American Journal of Surgery 175*, 367–370.

Duane, Therese, Wohlgemuth, Stephen, and Ruffin, Kirk MD, (2000) 'Intussusception After Roux-en-Y Gastric Bypass', *The American Surgeon 68*, 82–84.

'I'm A Whole New Woman' *Woman's World*, June 13, 2000.

Kirkpatrick, John R., and Zapas, John L. (1998) 'Divided Gastric Bypass: A Fifteen Year Experience', *The American Surgeon*

Kodama, K. (1998) 'Depressive Disorders as Psychiatric Complications After Obesity Surgery', *Psychiatry and Clinical Neuroscience 52*, 5 471–476.

Mason, E.E., (1998) 'Past, Present & Future of Obesity Surgery', *Obesity Surgery 8* 5, 524–529.

Moreno, Pau, Alastrue, Antoni, Rull, Miguel, Formeguera , Xavier, Casas, Dario, Boix, Jaume, Fernandez-Llamazares, Jaume, Broggi, Marc A. (1998) 'Band Erosion in Patients Who Have Undergone Vertical Banded Gastroplasty', *Archives of Surgery, 133*, Feb (1998) 'Laparoscopic Obesity Surgery Indications' 189–193.

Oria, H.E., and Brolin, R.E. (1999) 'Performance Standards in Bariatric Surgery', *European Journal of Gastroenterology and Hepatology 11* 2, 77–84.

Rand, C.S., Resnick, JL, and MacGregor, A.M. (1999) 'A Comparison of Body Size Evaluations Of Obesity Surgery Patients and General Population,' *Obesity Research 7,* 3 281–287.

Thornby, S.J., and Windsor, J.A. (1998) 'The Role of Surgery in the Management of Obesity,' *New Zealand Medical Journal 111,* 1078, November (1998), pp.445–448.

Wright, J. Kelly (1998) *Potential Benefits and Risks of Weight Loss Surgery.* Vanderbilt University Medical Center.

Useful Websites

www.nhlbi.nih.gov/guidelines/obesity/ob_home.htm
Published by the United States National Institutes of Health.
This website offers "Clinical Guidelines on the Identification,
Evaluation and Treatment of Overweight and Obesity in Adults".

www.obesity-online.com
Sponsored by Ethicon Endo-Surgery of Johnson and Johnson,
this site offers a variety of information and further references for
those interested in the treatment of obesity.

www.heartinfo.org/news97/obeshrt101597.htm
Highlighting publications on obesity from an international bank
of contributors, this site is maintained by the Center for
Cardiovascular Education, Inc. of New Providence, NJ, USA.

www.whyweight4success.com/favorite_links.htm
Provides direction toward organizations created to provide
assistance for weight control with emphasis on exercise,
motivation and help that is available. Privately maintained, this
site is a link resource for information.

**www.pbs.org/wgbh/pages/frontline/shows/fat/gateway
/surgery.html**
This site is produced as a public service by the National Institute
for Diabetic and Kidney Diseases and features a multidisciplinary
discussion of gastric surgery for obesity control.

www.surgicallyslim.com/links.htm
Created by Daniel M. Herron MD, this site serves to advertise the positive aspects of gastric surgery for obesity control but also provides linkage to several valuable non-advertising sites.

www.midwestsurgical.com/links.html
Presented by the American Surgical Obesity Institute, this is a linkage site that guides the reader to certification bodies and organizations of interest to those investigating the possibility of gastric surgery. Balancing pro and con, the site offers academic overviews from journal offerings to legal counsel.

www.beyondchange-obesity.com
Beyond Change offers a series of articles written in an easily readable format for those looking for additional information and varying viewpoints regarding obesity surgery.

www.mywls.com
This site is not only an explanatory vehicle but intersperses medical, surgical and dietary information with "before and after" pictures and testimonials from post-surgical patients. Privately maintained.

Index

Lightning Source UK Ltd.
Milton Keynes UK
UKOW03f0454120417
298922UK00001B/40/P